# Gina Explores Nature

## Lessons from a Magical Mat

**Traci Manuel**

Gina Explores Nature: Lessons from a Magical Mat

Traci Manuel

ISBN: 9781090231024

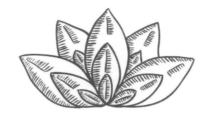

## Dedication

This book is dedicated to all the great yoga teachers that I have been privileged to practice with, as each one has inspired my journey in a meaningful way. One of particular note is Gina Gilligio, who impacted me in such a special way that I named the main character in this book Gina. Gina's raw honesty of her yoga path from practitioner to one of the most respected teachers has motivated me. She has also provided limitless support and guidance. BG So-honi, the character who is Gina's yoga class teacher, is of Indian descent. BG inspired me with his knowledge and teachings passed down from the great teachers who came before him. Finally, I would like to thank my husband who has not only been in full support of my yoga practice and this book, but every-thing I have interest in and endeavor to develop.

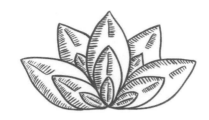

## Introduction

In the Western world, people sometimes think yoga is only for the uncommonly flexible or for practicing monks. In actuality, yoga has many different disciplines, making it accessible to people of all ages and capabilities. However today, kids are often over-scheduled by their parents from morning to night with school and various other activities. The idea of Gina's mat being magical and taking her to Nature, provided a vehicle to remove her from her overly busy young life, exacerbated by parental expectations. She and her mom get to travel to a place where she could learn yoga from animals and other elements of Nature. More importantly, both learn some powerful life lessons, which ultimately improve their already strained relationship. Read this book as parent and child together, or alone to capture the essence of yoga and learn some basic yoga poses along the journey.

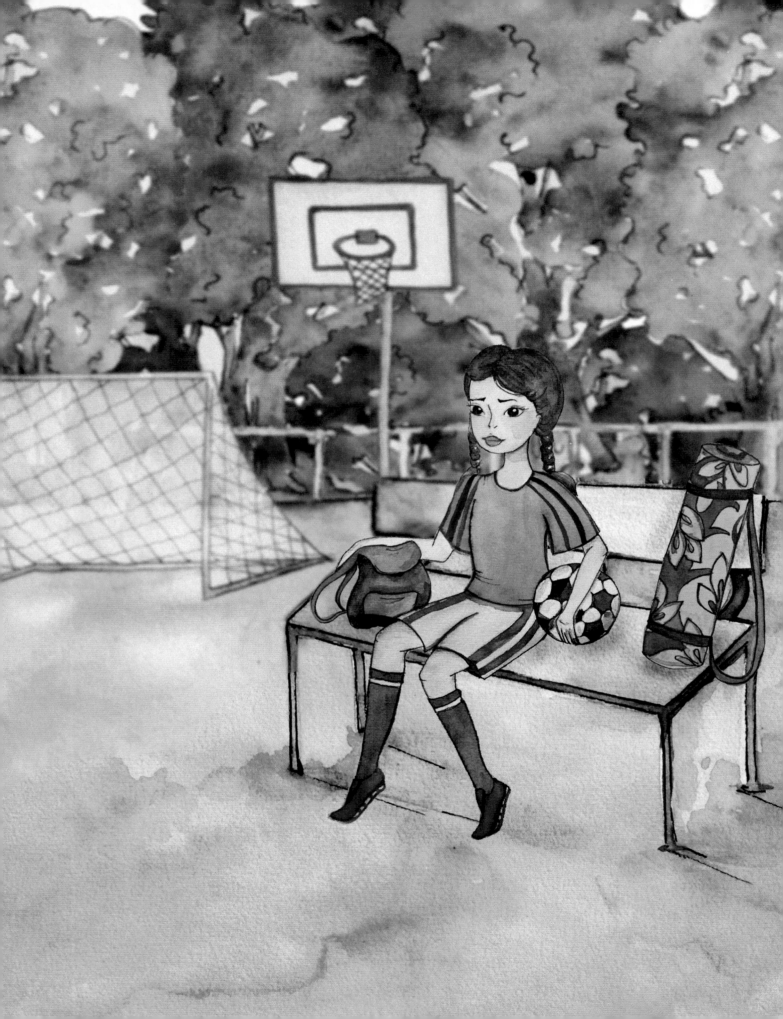

Gina sat on the bench at the soccer field waiting for her mom to arrive. They were going to yoga class together. Soccer practice had already started and it was Gina's second season. She really didn't want to join the team this year after a disappointing start last time. Instead, Gina longed to go to the park with her family on the weekends. Gina loved to color and in nature she would be able to find many different things to draw. Still, she often daydreamed of places far beyond her neighborhood. But now Gina, once again, was getting butterflies in her stomach. She sat, waiting nervously, while everyone else was picked up by their parents.

Gina was worried about yoga and wondering where her mom could be. Mom's goals for Gina were always different than her own. She thought yoga would help her become stronger and flexible, but Gina already had a jam-packed after-school schedule with soccer, ballet and gymnastics classes. At first, she wasn't sure if she would like yoga, but Gina wanted a chance to spend more time with her mom.

When Gina began yoga with her mom, she was allowed to pick out any mat from the different colors and styles at the studio. It was a tough choice, since there were so many gorgeous shades and patterns. Finally, she decided on the one she liked best - a pretty mat in grass green color with trees printed on it.

More important than all the new, fancy equipment was Gina's positive attitude. Gina started out with high hopes for enjoying her new activities, but once they began that all disappeared. Whether it was ballet, gymnastics, soccer, or even yoga, her parents would always push her to: pose perfectly, practice harder, win and score the most points. For Gina, this took all the fun out of her activities. Her early enthusiasm was squashed like a bug and for the most part she preferred to do something else, like stay home and color. All Gina really wanted was a sketchbook and crayons.

What's more, Mom always reminded Gina that they needed to arrive at class on time. But usually, her mom was the one running behind. She always got out of work late. Even on the weekends, she would frantically run errands and be short-tempered with Gina. Mom would feel rushed, and soon Gina would, too. Then came the butterflies...

Gina tried to do what BG the yoga teacher taught her when she felt them stirring inside. She would focus on her breath and think of things that made her happy. Her mind drifted to the park, spending time with family and drawing in nature. During recess, Gina would bring her crayons and sketch. At the park there was an infinite number of possibilities. With so many different species of birds, trees, flowers and creatures to draw, she'd never get bored!

Her thoughts were interrupted by the sound of Mom leaning on the horn. She jumped up, grabbed her bag and ran to the car.

As soon as she opened the door, she heard her mom saying, "Gina, you forgot your mat. Hurry, or we'll be late!" Gina ran back as quickly as she could and got into the car, fumbling as she locked the door and fastened her seatbelt. Mom nagged, "Were you daydreaming again? You're always forgetting things. Sometimes I think you would lose your head if it was not attached!" Gina was going to explain, but what was the point? Her mom never listened anyway. By the time Gina got to class she was upset and the butterflies had started again. BG always reminded his students that yoga gives us a chance to breathe, feel calm and happy. Gina thought that Mom must not remember this. Between working every day and taking Gina to all her activities, it seemed that Mom never had time to breathe.

As soon as they got on the road towards the studio, Mom asked, "Did you win? Did you score?" Mom usually started a conversation this way, asking about winning or losing, but not how Gina *enjoyed* the game. Gina began to answer, but Mom's phone rang. What was the use, anyway? She already felt her mom's disapproval heavy on her shoulders, like a cape weighing her down.

They sped through the parking lot and stuffed their coats and shoes into cubbies at the entrance to the studio. As soon as Gina entered the quiet room, she felt a soothing hush come over her body and she remembered to breathe deeply. Slowly she began to relax. Smelling like lavender, the room was warm and inviting. Even so, Mom interrupted her meditative state, "Gina, come on, we need to find a spot. Hurry up!"

Luckily, they entered the studio with a few moments to spare. Gina's mat made a loud slap on the smooth wooden floor. Everyone turned to look, frowning in their direction. Gina's face got hot and she started to sweat, even before beginning any of the poses. Everyone else was sitting quietly with their legs crossed in *Easy Seat (Sukhasana)*, waiting for BG the teacher to arrive.

Just as BG entered the room, Gina suddenly noticed a small caterpillar crawling on her Mom's mat and squealed.

"Ahh! Mom, look! There's a caterpillar on your mat. I'm scared. It's so hairy and ugly!"

Mom said, "Hush, Gina. BG's going to start. A caterpillar is small and can't hurt you. You have to get over your fears. Without caterpillars, we wouldn't have butterflies. Shh!" Gina loved butterflies, except the ones she had in her stomach, still fluttering around and around.

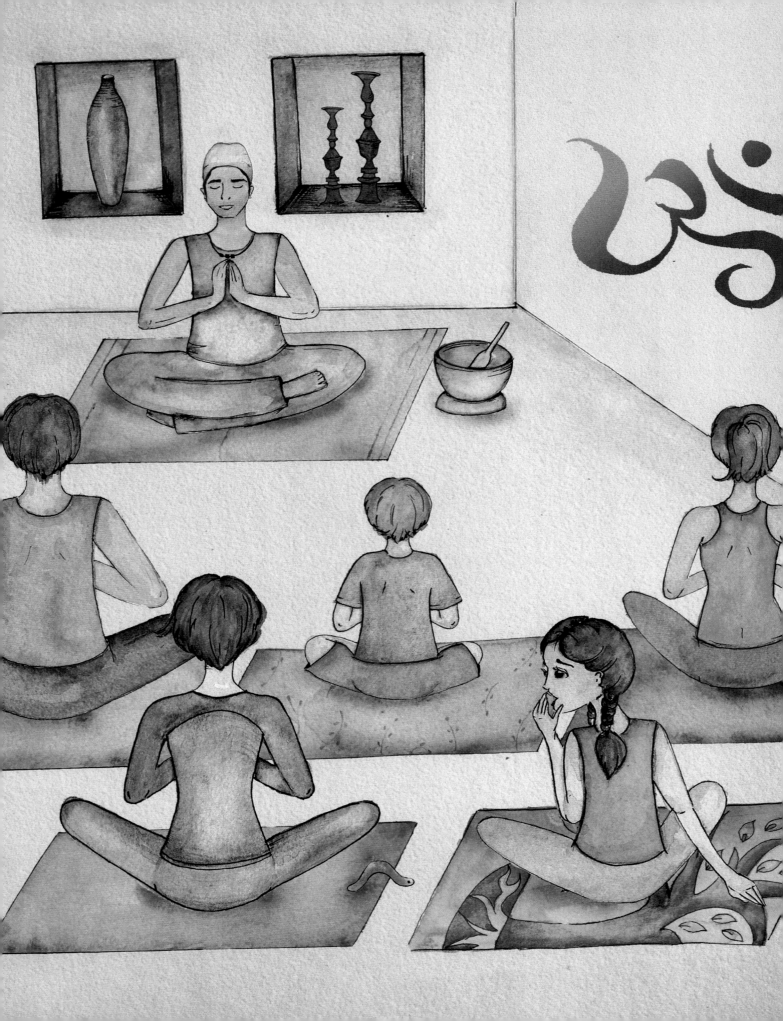

BG started, "*Namaste.*"

The class responded "*Namaste*" and pressed their hands together in front of their hearts in *Prayer Pose*, a position *called Anjali Mudra.* A mudra is a special symbol formed with hands to help focus in yoga class. Together they sang, "*Om Shanti! Shanti! Shanti! Peace! Peace! Peace!*" and class began. Then BG explained that now was the time to set an intention for their practice.

"What does that mean?" Gina wondered to herself.

BG answered, "An intention might be a few words to focus on, or a goal for to-day's practice. Maybe it's a positive saying you repeat in your head, or words of encouragement. For our class today I'd like us to think 'I am brave, I am calm. I don't fear change; I embrace it. Change brings growth.'"

"Hmm" Gina wondered to herself. "My intention for today is to be brave and not worry about those creepy caterpillars I'm so scared of. I just want to feel calm and get rid of these butterflies in my stomach once and for all! Oh, and not worry if my pose is right... Just have fun doing yoga!"

Gina tried not to pay attention to the caterpillar and instead focus on what BG was teaching. I guess he and Mom had a point. The caterpillar would even-tually change its gross form anyway and evolve into something beautiful.

Gina's mom considered BG's intention and took a fresh sip of air. Her idea was to fully let go of control and surrender to the practice. That would take bravery for sure. She had so many thoughts bombarding her, plus taking care of Gina and her brother, that her monkey mind was whirling non-stop.

During class, Gina's mom kept correcting her poses. Then again, she had done the same thing at the last class. In fact, Mom had been critiquing her practice ever since they started yoga together.

Gina slowly became very sad. She watched the other kids and their parents; it looked like they were having so much fun playing and laughing together. They would do poses like *Happy Baby Pose (Ananda Balasana)*, where they laid on their backs and grabbed their feet, rolling back and forth, bending their knees and pretending to walk on the ceiling. It looked like Gina's brother when he was an infant - he used to latch onto his toes and roll around in his crib just like that.

Meanwhile, Gina could not even learn this most basic, natural *asana* (pose) with her mom constantly trying to fix her.

Gina was eagerly awaiting the final pose of the class. This was her favorite part because during Resting Pose (*Savasana*) Gina could actually relax. She couldn't wait for her mom to stop nagging her and just lie down and be still. Here she could recline on her mat, heart up to the sky, hands open and eyes closed. She'd take a big inhale, let go and feel her body sink into the mat. All the butterflies she had at the beginning of class seemed to float away and she felt light and relaxed, almost like she was floating on a cloud.

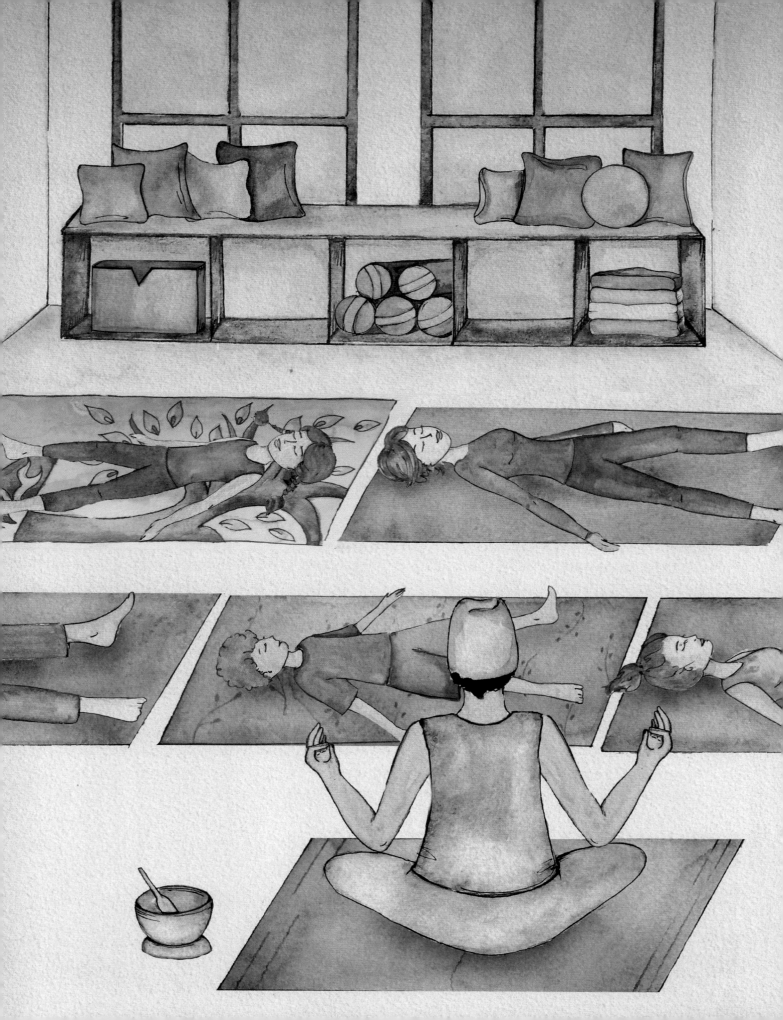

At first, this pose was difficult since her mind would drift. Gina wanted to jump off her mat as her imagination bombarded her with ideas of things to draw. But BG reminded everyone to try and not think of anything during this do-nothing pose. "Just be", he said.

Sometimes it was hard not to drift away completely. The lights were dimmed, soft music was playing from the speakers overhead and candles flickered in the sweet-smelling studio. Gina was exhausted from all her running and rushing. She placed one hand on her chest and felt her heart beating, calm and steady. Usually she laid still in *Savasana* without falling asleep, yet today her eyes felt heavy and started to close. Gina surrendered completely to the floor and, before she knew it, she had fallen fast asleep.

The relaxing music BG played started to sound farther and farther away. Gina started to dream that her yoga mat lifted off the ground where she was supposed to be just resting, doing nothing. On the mat, her mom was sitting next to her as the mat took off in flight. She felt her yoga mat lift off the floor and leave the solid earth beneath her.

Gina squealed gleefully, "Mom, how did you get here? This is so exciting! I had no idea that the mat we picked out could actually fly. Can you hold my hand? I'm a little scared. You know I'm afraid of heights."

Her mom looked stern. "Gina, you're a big girl now! You are nine years old, almost ten. There's no reason to be afraid. Just hold onto the sides of your mat. You know they are called 'sticky mats' for a reason. It's safe. Be brave."

Gina listened to her mom and gripped the sides of her mat as tightly as she could. They soared through the sky, circling around beautiful clouds, heading higher and higher until they were nearly to the sun! They traveled on their magical mat for a long time until night fell and the moon and stars filled the sky.

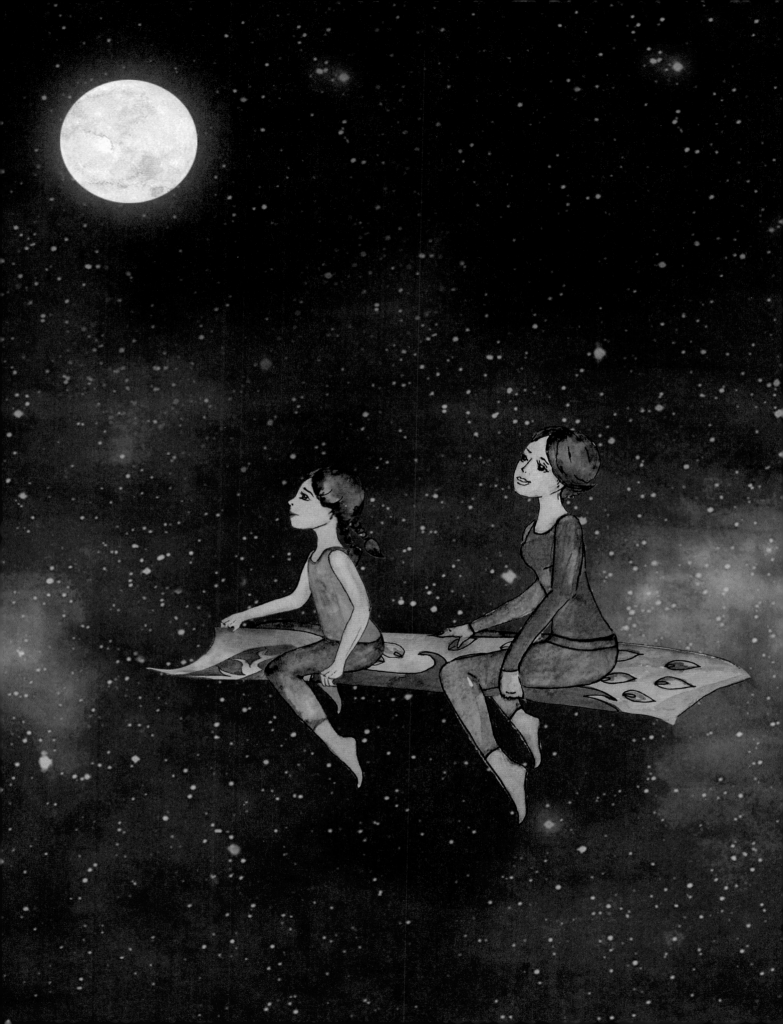

Finally, as the moon disappeared and the sun began to rise, the mat descended towards a green and luscious place. Gina and her mom landed in a beautiful valley full of mountains, trees, rivers and flowers. It was more breathtaking than Gina could ever imagine!

They climbed off the mat and looked around. Gina couldn't believe how tall the trees were. She tried to count the branches, but lost track as she noticed how small they seemed against the huge mountains standing behind them. The river stretched out into the distance, never-ending and the valley floor was filled with the most brilliant flowers she had ever seen.

Gina's eyes widened as they took in all the splendid sights surrounding them. Gina's big brown eyes grew wider still, sparkling with wonder and delight.

"Namaste" a voice called out from above in the treetops.

"Who is that?" Gina asked, looking all around, her brown eyes growing bigger yet!

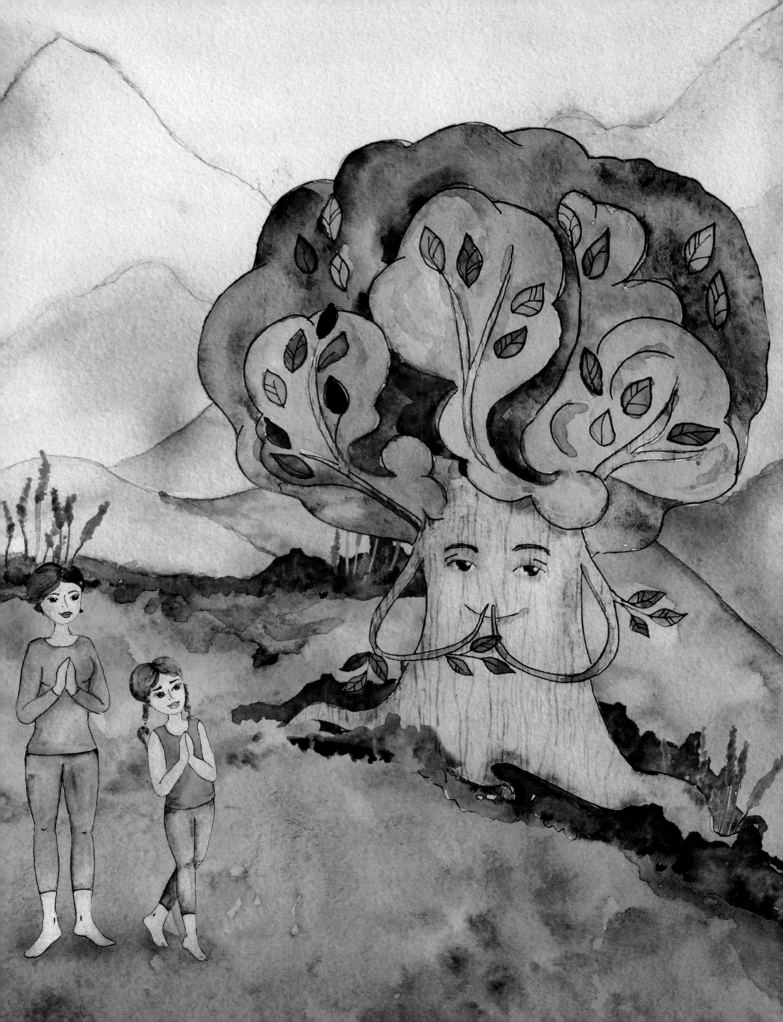

"Namaste. It is me", Tyler the Tree said as he bowed his head and pressed his branches together at heart center. It reminded Gina of how her teacher BG would fold his hands in prayer at the beginning and end of every class.

"I saw something flying through the sky above my branches. I was unsure of what it was. I knew it wasn't a plane or a star. Then I saw you land in our valley on that pretty green mat! I had no idea yoga mats could fly. It must be magical. Welcome! I am Tyler the Tree. What are your names?"

"Namaste" the pair replied in unison and bowed their heads to Tyler, hands at heart center.

"I am Gina and this is my mom Elizabeth. I picked out this mat to do yoga with my mom. I didn't know it could fly either! Where are we? What is this amazing place we've landed in?" Gina asked curiously.

Tyler replied, "You are here in Nature. My friends and I all work together in living harmony. See all the other trees rooted into the ground beside me? The mountains stand firm behind me, the flowers reach their blossoms to the sun overhead, the birds fly high in the sky and those that rest on my branches, all animals on land and sea - we are all Nature. We have so many friends. Not only big creatures, but small critters too like the butterflies and the bees. The stars, the moon, the sun and the planets are all a part of this peaceful space called Nature."

"How do you know the word *Namaste*, Tyler?" asked Gina.

"*Namaste* is the way we have greeted one another in Nature for thousands of years. By greeting one another we honor each other, just as you - a budding young yogi, your mom and your fellow yogis - do in class. This is the way of Nature. We have practiced yoga since time began. Now, tell me about yourselves. We rarely have visitors drop in from the sky on a magical ride! Where are you from?" Tyler asked.

Gina replied, "We live in the City. It has a lot of tall buildings, streets full of beeping cars in traffic and many people rushing around, bumping into each other. It is not nearly as quiet as your home here. Mom, see how quiet and peaceful it is here in Nature? This is why I'm always asking to go to the park with you and Dad."

Gina's mom looked as if she was listening, but didn't reply. Gina turned again to Tyler. "Tyler, you are so tall. I lost track of counting all your branches. I feel so small beside you."

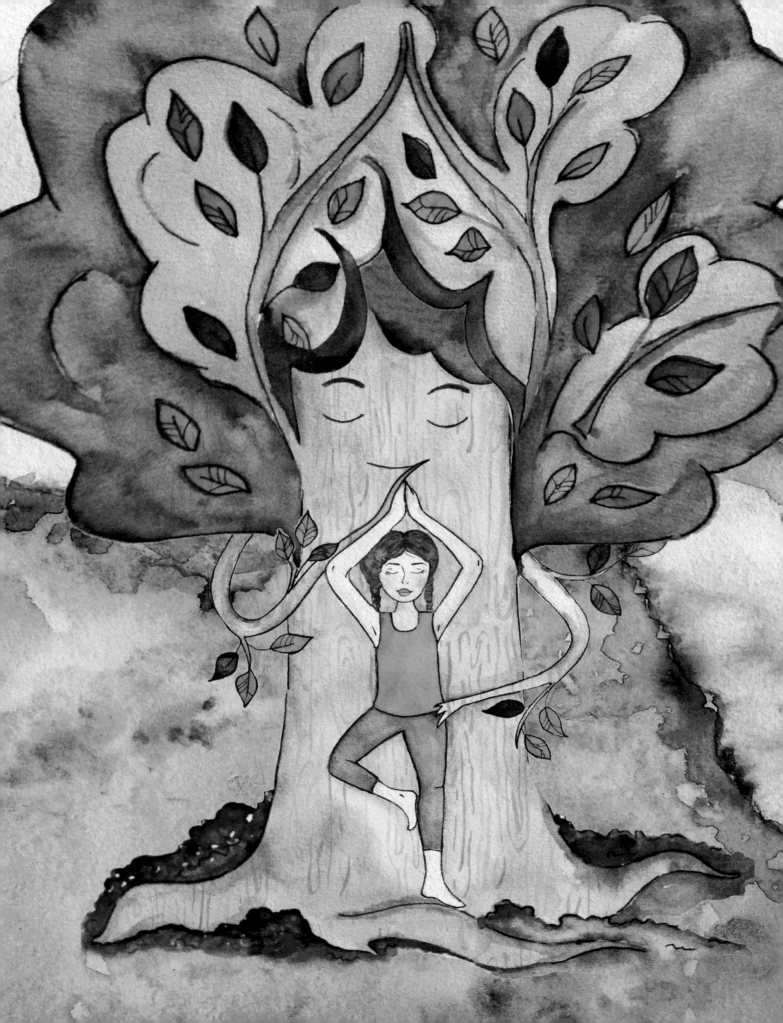

Tyler said, "Come stand right next to me, Gina. I want to show you *Tree Pose (Vrksasana)*. Stand up tall, rooting both feet into the ground and feel Mother Earth's floor pushing back to support you. Just like we trees depend on the Earth for stability, you too can grow strong by connecting to her floor. Find a spot to focus on; it could be a rock or a log, something that won't move. This will help you steady yourself. Now raise your leg and bend your knee. Rest your foot against your standing leg on your ankle or above your knee. Then you will be balancing on one leg like me. This *asana* helps develop focus and determination, which you need in everything you do in life. Lift your arms to the sky and spread your fingers apart like my branches. Grow as tall as you can. Connect all corners of your feet into the earth to root down, then rise up even higher. You might sway the way my branches move in the wind, or you may remain perfectly still like on a hot summer day. Remember, your standing leg creates a strong foundation. This shows you how to be flexible, but also strong at the same time, just like a tree" Tyler explained.

Gina tried to do as Tyler explained. Just like in class, after a few times of falling over, she could stand on one leg and raise her arms to the sky with Tyler helping her.

Tyler told Gina that trees are very patient creatures and live a long time. Like a tree, Gina can choose to practice patience while balancing the many choices in life. There is no rush. Her ability and wishes will change over time just as trees' leaves change throughout the seasons.

Gina thanked Tyler and said, "This makes me feel so happy. I love trees. I bet you can tell from looking at my mat! Now it will always remind me of you, Tyler."

Tyler smiled. "You can practice standing like a tree whenever you want to feel happy and balanced. Once you get tired, you can slide your foot down slowly and lower your arms to your sides with your heart wide open and your gaze up toward the sky, smiling at the sun. Then you'll be posing in *Mountain Pose (Tadasana)*, like Marc the Mountain, who stands majestically behind me. Hey Marc, we have some new friends that came to visit. They just arrived here in Nature from the City."

"Namaste," Marc the Mountain called out. "It's so nice to have you visit our valley. You arrived at the perfect time while the sun is beginning to rise. We like to salute the sun every morning as it appears, giving gratitude for the new day. We honor the warmth and light that the sun provides. What are you grateful for?"

"Hmm" thought Gina. "Today I am thankful to have my mom with me on this journey, to meet new friends in Nature and explore a different place." Gina felt her body warm with happiness as she thought of all the positive things happening in her life.

"Feel free to climb up to my peak. From up here you have a spectacular view!" called Marc.

Gina replied, "I'm afraid of heights. Even flying on the magic mat, I was so scared. Mom said at my age I shouldn't be afraid, but I still am."

Marc said, "If you want to try, go slowly and breathe with each step you take. If you are brave and face your fear, you may be able to overcome it. If you focus on your breathing and the steady Earth beneath you, you'll feel peaceful. You will always be supported and safe within our mountain range. Or you can stand here right beside me and practice *Sun Salutations (Surya Namaskar)*. Raise your arms up overhead. Connect your palms together and gaze up at the Sky."

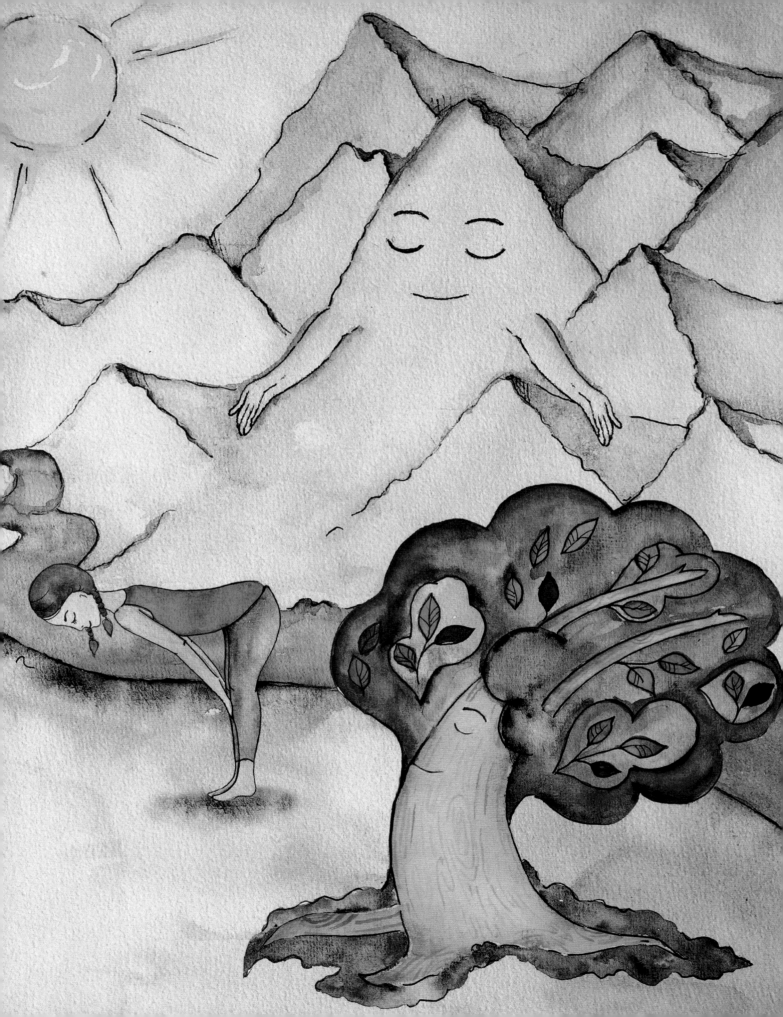

"If you don't mind, I think I'll stay here for now," Gina said, a bit bashfully. Then she grew taller as she swept her arms above her and the sun beamed on her face. She smiled and closed her eyes to feel its warm rays.

Marc spoke kindly. "That's fine Gina. You look great." He turned to Gina's mom and asked, "Elizabeth, how would you like to climb up?"

Elizabeth smiled sheepishly. "I'd prefer to stay down here, next to Gina."

Gina looked over at her mom with surprise. "Mom, are you afraid of heights, too?"

"No," Elizabeth replied a bit too quickly, "I would rather stay here. I'm feeling tired from the long day of travel."

Gina suggested they all take a short rest in *Child's Pose (Balasana)*. Gina and her mom folded their chests over bent knees and softened onto their ankles. Gina walked her fingers out in front of her like a spider, stretching her arms nice and long. Gina's mom took a different variation, bringing her hands behind her head in prayer. Marc slowly lowered down and allowed his peak to touch the ground, since he usually stands all day. Tyler extended his branches towards his roots instead of holding them up high. Everyone took a nice break and sighed out in relief, enjoying the chance to rest.

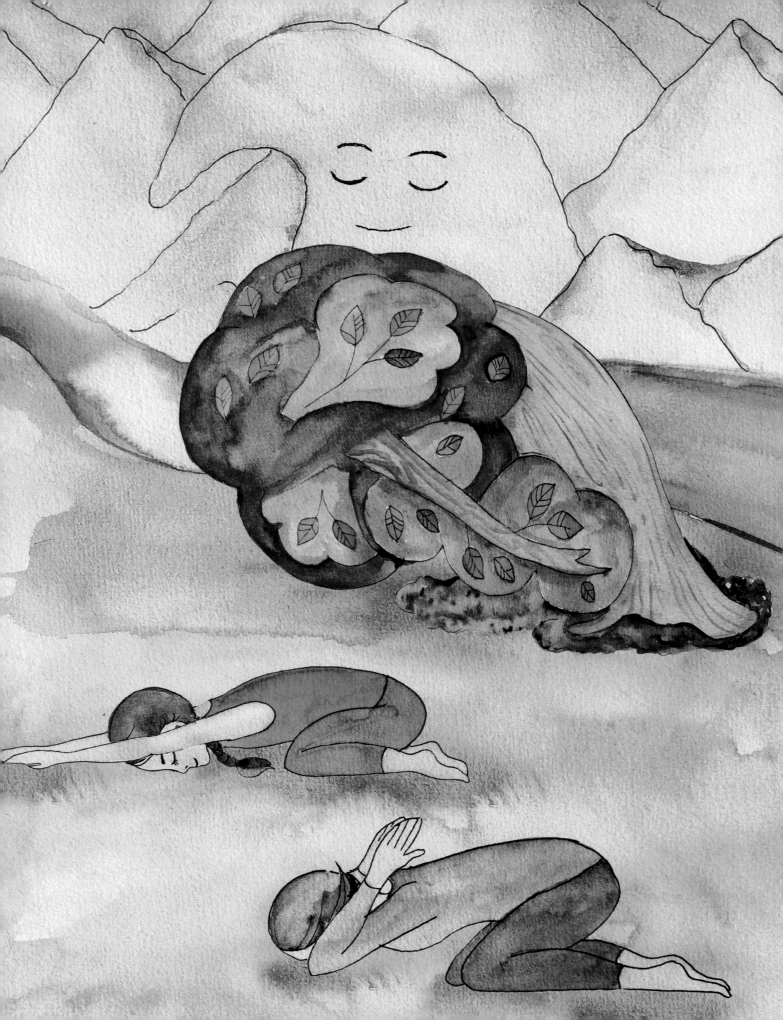

Gina shifted closer to her mom and asked, "Mom, when you were my age, were you ever afraid of heights?"

"No," she answered. "I never was, which is why I hope you can overcome your fear soon. There's nothing to be afraid of."

Marc saw how Gina suddenly looked very sad from what her mom said. He reminded Gina, "Whenever you do feel fear, focus on breathing deeply. That may help you calm down and feel less afraid."

Gina said, "Marc, I'll try. I often get scared not only of heights, but when I have competitions with a large audience of people watching, even Mom and Dad. I know I should feel proud that they are coming to see me perform, but I get so worried about letting them down in front of everyone."

Gina's eyes welled up with tears. She tried to swipe at them quickly so no one would see her crying, but it was too late. Marc noticed the tears rolling down her cheeks. He reassured Gina that there was no need for her to climb his mountains if she did not want to. When and if she was ready, he would always be there for her, strong and steady.

"Gina," Marc blurted out, "you are perfect as you are right now in the present moment. In fact, you remind me of the Goddess of Nature herself."

"The Goddess of Nature?" Gina repeated. "Who is the Goddess of Nature? What does she look like?"

Marc looked a bit shy as he replied, "The Goddess of Nature was the prettiest girl in Nature." Then he could say no more. He did not remember her well, since she lived there many, many years ago.

Marc suddenly called out to Eli the Elephant who was grazing in a meadow beyond Tyler and the other trees in the valley.

Marc explained that elephants, besides being the strongest mammals, have an excellent memory.

"Eli, you have the best memory of us all. Can you tell our new friends what you remember about the Goddess of Nature?"

Eli swayed slowly over to where Gina and her mom were talking to Marc and Tyler. Neither had ever seen an elephant outside the zoo.

Gina noticed that Eli was walking on the tips of his toes. "Mom, look at Eli! He is tip-toeing like humans do when we want to be quiet. Did you know they walk this way?"

Her mom answered, "Yes, Gina. It's what you and your brother do when you sneak out of bed early. I didn't know that elephants do that though."

Gina exclaimed, "Mom, how did you know that? Next time we tiptoe, I will remember that I am walking like an elephant. We can learn so much here in Nature."

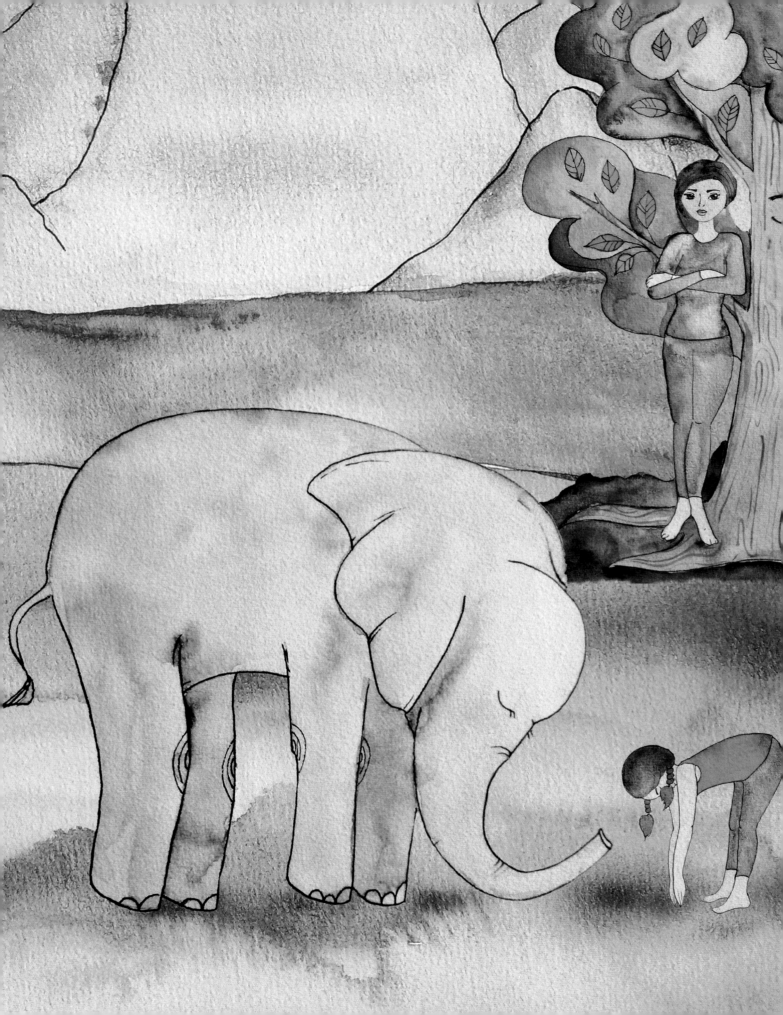

Gina tried to pose like Eli in *Elephant Pose ( Gaja Vadivu)* by bending over. The trunk of her body hung down. She stood on the tips of her toes as her fingertips grazed the grass. Then she toppled over her heels and landed gently on the soft ground.

Gina, Marc, Eli and Tyler all started to laugh. Elizabeth, however, did not crack even a thin smile. She looked impatient as Gina quickly got up and dusted off her new yoga outfit.

Eli said, "Namaste, Gina and welcome. The Goddess of Nature was beautiful as Marc described, especially when she laughed, just like you! She reminded us that little girls can do whatever they wish! They can use their imagination and dress-up, or roll in the grass and do sports too. They certainly love to giggle and are very strong indeed."

Eli continued, swinging his trunk for emphasis as he spoke. "The Goddess used to stand with her feet wide, strong and steady, while her toes and knees pointed out, open towards the valley. Her heels faced each other and she bent her knees. She was strong and rooted to the Earth. She would raise her arms towards the clouds and keep her balance. Or, sometimes she folded them in prayer, closed her eyes and smiled. We call this position *Goddess Pose (Utkata Konasana)* to honor her. She was not only beautiful, but also the kindest woman in Nature. She stood out amongst the other maidens living here. She was not prickly, like Carol the Cactus over there."

Eli raised his trunk and pointed it to a large cactus in the distance. Gina asked Eli, "Why is Carol so prickly?"

Eli replied, "Instead of leaves, cacti have spiny needles that help them store water. This adaptation protects them from thirsty animals that would try to nibble them. It's not Carol's fault - after all, it is her natural state. But like her spiny needles, she would often hurt animals by accident through her actions and words. She forgets to breathe and then reacts with whatever's on her mind. We all must remember to calm down first, breathe deeply and center our mind and body before acting. Then we won't cause harm.

Eli looked at Gina standing before him. "Gina, try Goddess Pose like I explained before. I would show you how, but my legs don't move like that. In yoga, everyone's poses might look different and that's okay. Even the teacher may not know how to do everything, but we can always help one another with our practice. There's no such thing as perfect. That's why we call it a *practice*."

Gina placed her feet in a wide line and pivoted her heels in as Eli had explained. Suddenly, a big smile came across her face. "Look, this is easy! This *asana* reminds me of the pliés we do in ballet! Look Mom, this is how the Goddess of Nature stood! If I bend down even lower, I squat like that frog over by the river! This must be how they get power in their legs to jump so far."

Elizabeth didn't look impressed. "See Gina, I told you learning ballet is important for proper posture."

Marc spoke, "Gina, not only are you a talented ballerina, you are also a fine young yogi. You really remind me so much of the Goddess of Nature. Do you mind if we call you Gina the Goddess?"

This time Gina was blushing. She murmured, "I don't know. I'm sure she was much prettier than me."

"Nonsense!" hooted Oscar the Owl, who had been silently watching everything while perched comfortably on Tyler's branch.

Gina and Elizabeth both turned to look up. There high above them sat Oscar. They had been so busy learning new things that they did not notice he had flown in and was watching over the gathering of friends.

He blinked his big, yellow eyes at them slowly as he spoke. "Beauty comes from the inside. It lives in your heart and soul, like the kindness Eli mentioned. It's not just on the outside; it is a light that shines from within. We say *Namaste* to each other to honor the beauty in all beings. Gina, it is obvious you have both inner *and* outer beauty. You deserve to be called Gina the Goddess here and wherever you go."

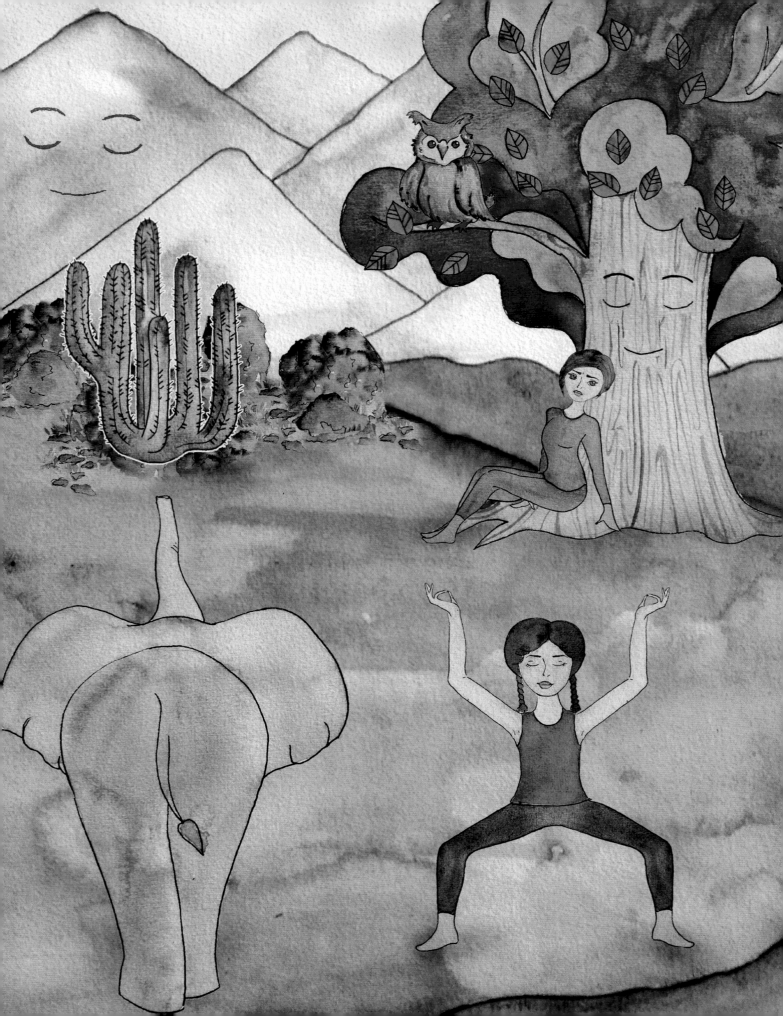

Marc grinned. "Well, that's settled then. Goddess Gina! There's no sense in arguing with Oscar. You probably know that owls are among the wisest birds on Earth. Not only that, they can turn their heads very far around. Elizabeth, do you know how far an owl can turn his head?"

Elizabeth looked stumped. "Nope. Maybe 180 degrees, half-way?" Oscar demonstrated by turning his head almost full circle. "Oh, my goodness", Elizabeth exclaimed with curiosity and admiration in her voice.

"Wow!" Gina shouted, "I never noticed this before! It kind of looks like how we do neck rolls and relax our shoulders at the beginning of class with BG".

"You're right!" her mom responded in awe. "I never knew this about owls. It's really neat!"

Suddenly, Gina and her mom exchanged a new look. Something in their eyes shone in a different way, showing curiosity and respect. Gina looked away shyly.

Then she stared down at her bare feet and asked, "Mom, can we go to the park more often and learn about the things here in Nature?"

"Perhaps" her Mom replied slowly. "Right now, between yoga, ballet and gymnastics..." Elizabeth stared off anxiously into space. She took a deep breath then looked steadily at Gina. "It's not the right time. Maybe in a few weeks when school is out during summer vacation."

But Gina couldn't wait for summer. She knew there was so much to learn in Nature. She looked back at Oscar and tried to mimic him and see how far her head could turn. Gina started posing like an owl by squatting on her heels and twisting her upper body and head one direction, and then the other. Again, all the friends started to laugh, everyone except Elizabeth. She still looked so serious.

"Elizabeth," Oscar said, "it's wonderful to hear that Gina is involved in so many activities involving exercise! This will keep her strong in body and mind. Walking in the park, hiking up mountains like Marc, practicing balance beneath a tree like Tyler or standing strong like the Goddess herself are all important. Plus, when you exercise outdoors, the whole experience is even better! Breathing in fresh air and looking at the beautiful forms of life around us are as important as all the busywork that takes place indoors. Being outside activates all your senses. It makes you feel at one with Nature."

Oscar turned to Gina and asked her, "Gina do you know how many senses we have?"

Gina raised her hand up with five fingers showing, and yelled out, "Five!" She then counted them off on one finger at a time, "sight, sound, taste, touch and smell."

Tyler nodded, impressed. "By using our senses in Nature, we learn things that help us every day. Just observe the world around you! Close your eyes and smell the pines. Listen for the calling of birds on the opposite side of the valley. Savor the richness of fruit picked right off the tree, or feel the smoothness of a stone, perfect for skipping on the water. Indoor activities like chores and homework are necessary, yes - but outdoors you can explore and be creative! You must try new things and learn to adapt to the circumstances. For instance, if a rainstorm is coming, you can observe the clouds and listen for thunder. Nature gives us warning signals so we can avoid danger. We may need to take different routes and change our plans to avoid floods and return safely."

"See Mom? We can learn so much from Nature and our surroundings. That's why I'm always begging you to go to the park", Gina explained.

The new friends were so busy getting to know each other they forgot about food. Tyler exclaimed, "Forgive me for not being a better host! I didn't offer you something to eat! Please take a banana from its tree, or any fruit growing here. Gently pick whichever snack you like and come down by the river where we can all sit and feast."

Gina and Elizabeth each selected a ripe banana and made their way down the path to the river. Gina saw a big tiger sprawled out over the rocks, arching and lowering his back a few times. It pressed its paws into the rock as it curled its spine and bowed its head. Then it reversed the movement and opened its heart to the sky, lifting its tail and raising its gaze up towards the sun. Suddenly the tiger let out a big roar and Gina jumped.

Tyler yelled out to Tommy the Tiger. "Hey Tommy, no need to show off with that big roar! We have some new visitors and you are scaring Gina." Gina turned red. Tyler introduced Gina to Tommy.

She was nervous about walking on the rocks towards the water. But she saw the river was filled with beautiful pink and white flowers and wanted to see them up close so she could sketch them later. Tommy, showing that his roar was bigger than his bite, invited Gina to walk on his strong back like a bridge over the running river.

Tommy explained to her that he kept his back strong and flexible doing those movements. Gina mentioned, "This reminds me of *Cat-Cow Pose (Bitilasana-Marjaryasana)* I learned!" Tyler offered to hold her hand as Tommy carried her across. As a team, they successfully crossed the river. Gina felt safe with Tommy guiding her and Tyler's outstretched branch supporting her.

Gina asked, "What type of flower is that, Oscar? I know you are wise in the ways of Nature."

Before Oscar could even answer, a voice yelled out, "A lotus! Everyone here in Nature knows the beauty and grace of the lotus."

Gina's pink face showed her embarrassment.

"Charlie the Crocodile, you should be ashamed of yourself," Marc scolded. "These are our guests and you are being cranky as always." Marc smiled broadly at Gina and Elizabeth. "I apologize for our friend Charlie. Sometimes we call him 'Cranky Charlie' and you can see why! He has a personality like Carol."

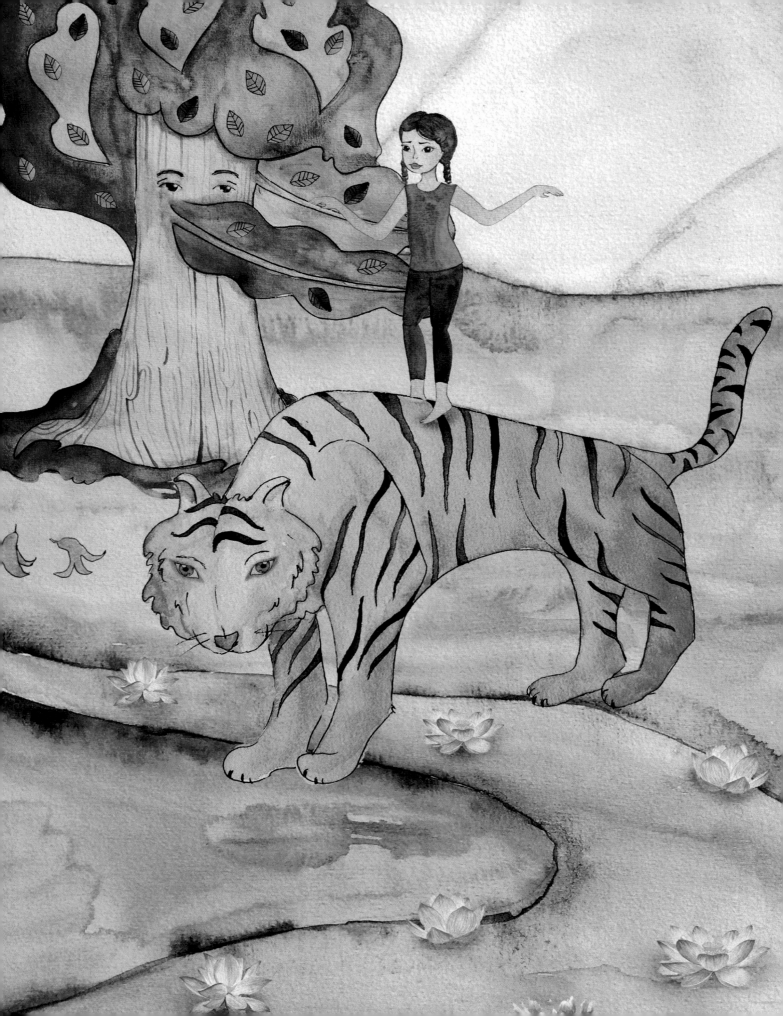

Oscar told Gina how lotus flowers bloom in the day and sink below the water at night, closing tight like a fist. "Then they rise to open their petals again the next morning. They root in the muck and mud, but grow towards the light, sparkling to the surface. This shows us that even if we find ourselves in a tough situation or are having a bad day, each morning we can choose to start fresh and rise up, shining like the sun, brand-new."

Oscar taught Gina and Elizabeth the way to make *Lotus Seal (Padma Mudra)* with their hands and to sit in *Lotus Pose (Padmasana)*. To start, they both sat with their legs crossed and their spines nice and straight. Next, they brought their wrists together and connected their thumbs with one another and then their pinky fingers. This made a special bowl from which they spread their petal-like fingers and let them open and close. Gina closed her eyes as she lifted her Lotus upwards like the flowers do when they float on the surface. Oscar mentioned, "In *Lotus Pose (Padmasana)*, every breath you take opens your chest and heart to blossom even more fully."

Gina pointed out a butterfly that had just perched itself on a petal of the lotus. "Look everyone, there's a butterfly! Her wings are big and they move so fast with so many bright and beautiful colors."

Oscar said, "Now uncross your legs. Put the soles of your feet together in *Butterfly Pose (Baddha Konasana)* and pump your knees up and down. See? Your legs move like butterfly wings in this pose." Gina giggled in delight, feeling the movements of her legs to be graceful like the flapping of a butterfly.

While Gina fluttered her legs, Elizabeth looked out along the river's edge. Charlie slithered up the riverbank to apologize. Charlie could be very grouchy and snappy, but he was also a charmer and sweet as could be. Big crocodile tears now rolled down his cheeks. Honestly, he never wanted to hurt anyone's feelings.

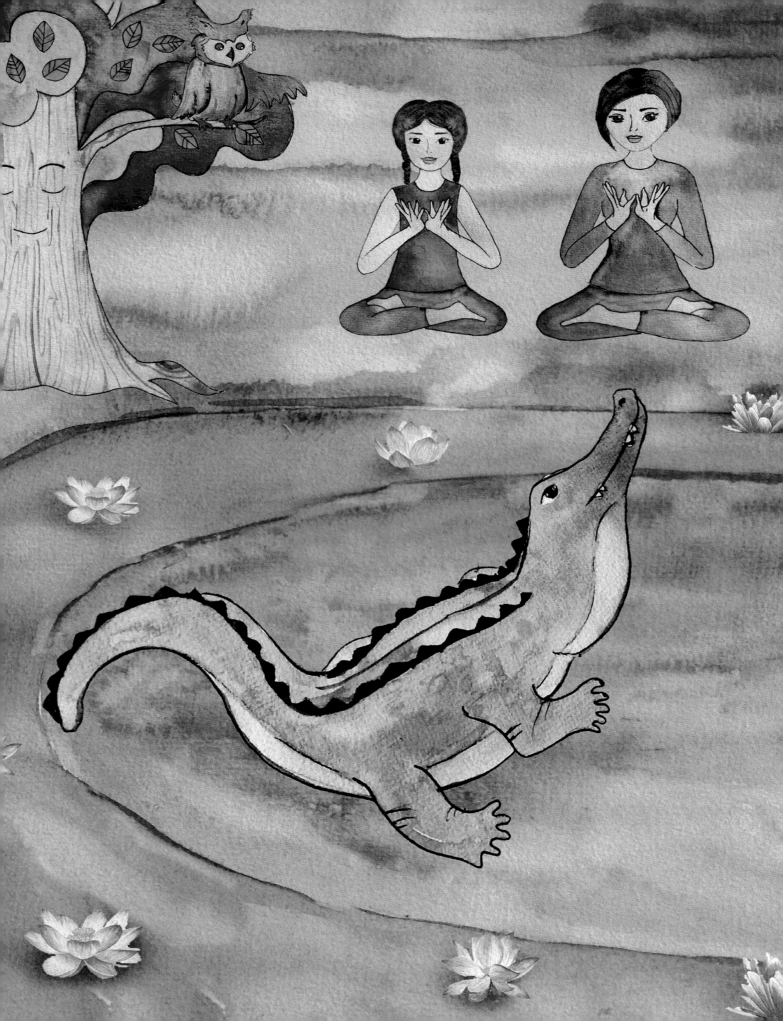

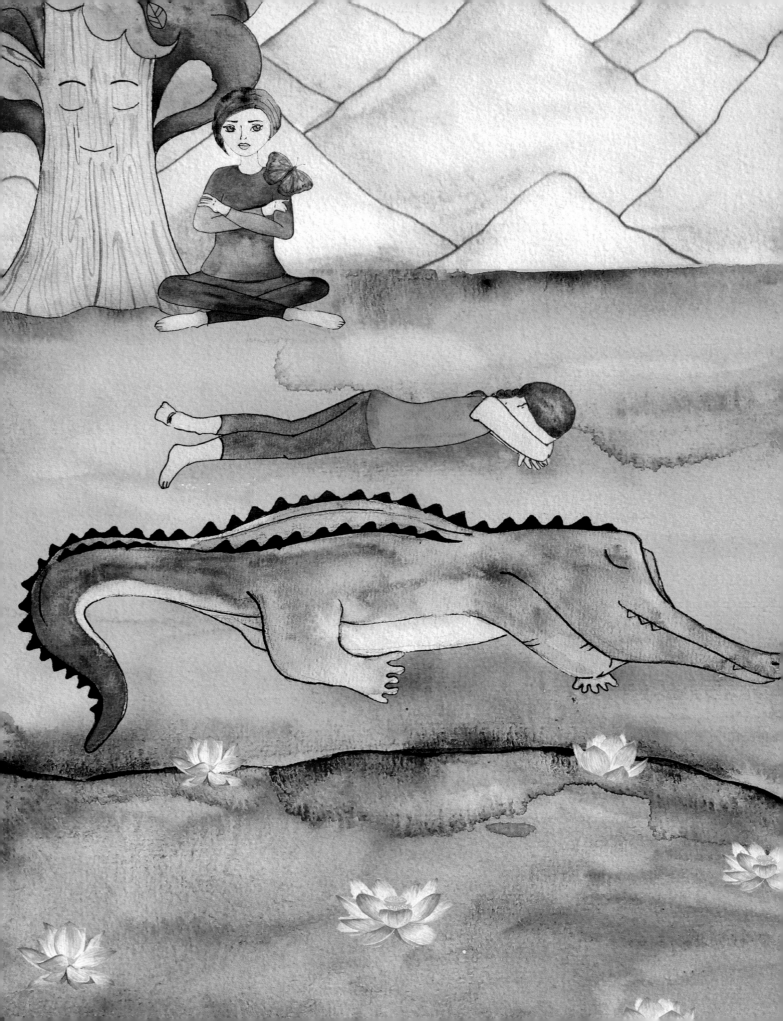

Gina knew Charlie was caring and gentle. She unfolded her legs and lay down next to Charlie, putting her arm around him. She tried to extend just as he was stretched long from head to tail. She lay on her stomach with her feet hip width apart, toes pointing inward and heels facing out. She folded her arms in front of her and rested her head on her hands in *Crocodile Pose (Makarasana)*. She told Charlie she loved to lie like him at home when she colored. Coloring, she explained, was her favorite activity, but she did not have a lot of free time with all the activities she has. Then she accepted Charlie's apology and knew deep down he had a kind heart.

Just then the butterfly flew from the lotus petal and landed on Elizabeth's shoulder where she was watching the scene unfolding before her with a gentle gaze.

"Mom, look! The butterfly is on your shoulder! You know, even though I'm afraid of small hairy caterpillars, when they transform into beautiful butterflies they become so different... not scary. I like them much better when they are flying in Nature than in my stomach!" Everyone laughed except for Elizabeth. Gina tried to get her mom to lighten up. She noticed, "Mom, this butterfly is a combination of your favorite colors. Look at the gorgeous purple, red and black designs on her wings. She reminds me of you."

After, Tyler asked if anyone knew three things a crocodile and an owl have in common.

Marc observed Charlie's tears and guessed they both cry. Eli remembered they both lay eggs, but could not think of a third shared trait. Gina shouted, "I know! We just learned this in school. They both have excellent night vision."

"Very wise, Goddess Gina, now let's see if you know the answer to this last riddle. What do Charlie the Crocodile and Eli the Elephant have in common?"

Gina said, "That's simple! They are both among the strongest animals on earth!"

Oscar looked pleased. "Right again! Gina, what's this? Are you trying to snap up my job as the wisest being in Nature? I better sharpen my skills now that you're with us!"

As they all giggled, Gina peeked over at her mom. Even Elizabeth was laughing this time!

Elizabeth stopped laughing, but her face looked relaxed and peaceful. She had been unusually quiet for a long while. Gina noticed she seemed to have a glow around her. She shone with an inner wisdom as she turned to face the group of friends.

Elizabeth finally spoke. "Oscar, Tyler, I have been thinking all this time about what you have been saying." All the friends looked intently as Elizabeth continued. "My own mom, Gina's grandmother, takes a walk outside every day and is very healthy. She works, but also makes time to relax. She goes to the park to walk and even plays tennis with her friends. Sadly, my dad, never exercised much and is unhealthy now. In fact, he's quite ill and everyone is so worried about him. One day he seemed fine and the next thing you know, he was very sick."

Elizabeth continued, her voice growing stronger as she shared her story. "You see, Gina's grandfather spent his days working hard and never taking time to relax. He worked to give his family everything and never once thought of his own health. We didn't encourage him to do other activities because he was always strong and proud. We didn't want to hurt his feelings because he worked so hard for us. But you make a good point. Being outside is good for our health and helps us learn to enjoy the present moment. We must take breaks, go outside and breathe deeply. Then we can return to our work and feel calmer and better doing it."

Elizabeth seemed very thoughtful as she spoke and smiled. Gina noticed a faraway look in her eyes that reminded her of daydreaming. Her mom looked lost in deep thought.

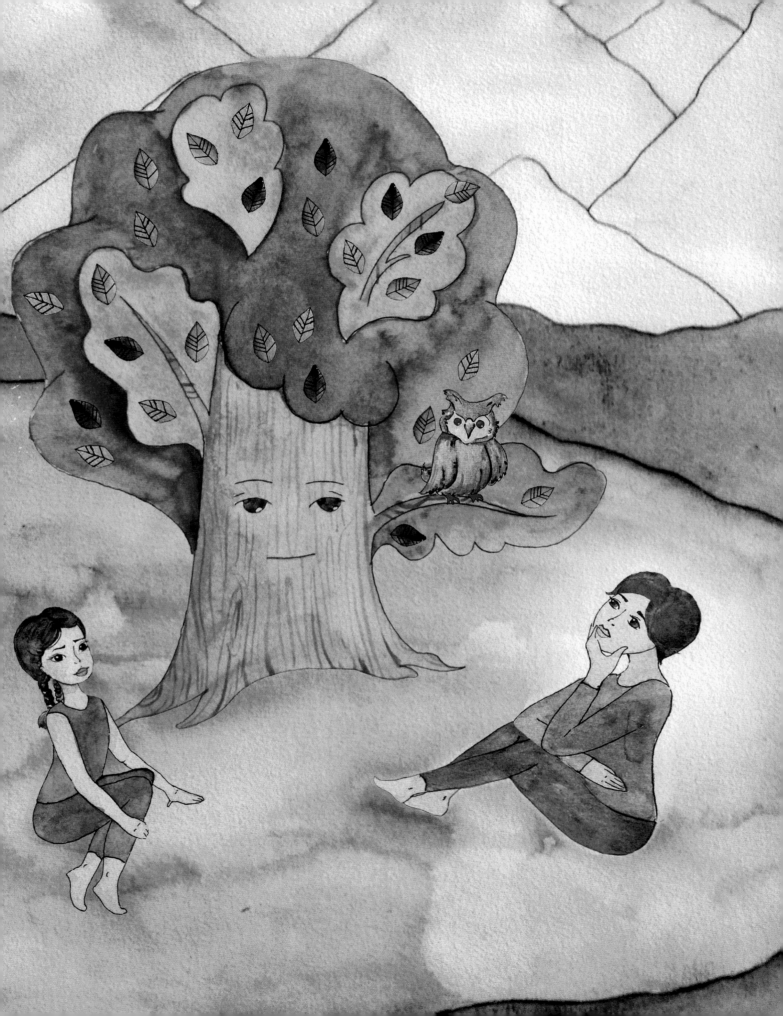

Oscar, very satisfied with Elizabeth's comment, let out a big "HOO HOO!" to show his agreement. This startled Elizabeth who jumped and then laughed. Gina answered back, "HOO! HOO!" Then everyone was laughing and calling out, Elizabeth the loudest of all.

Gina, feeling very happy, lay down next to Charlie to show him *Happy Baby Pose, (Ananda Balasana)*. She instructed him to rollover on his back, grab his hind feet with his front limbs and rock from side to side. "It's like a nice massage for your scales!" she said. Charlie used his tail to find his balance and he swayed back and forth, letting the sun warm his belly. All the day's movements tired Gina out. She was already feeling quite sleepy. She lay her head down and rested next to Charlie.

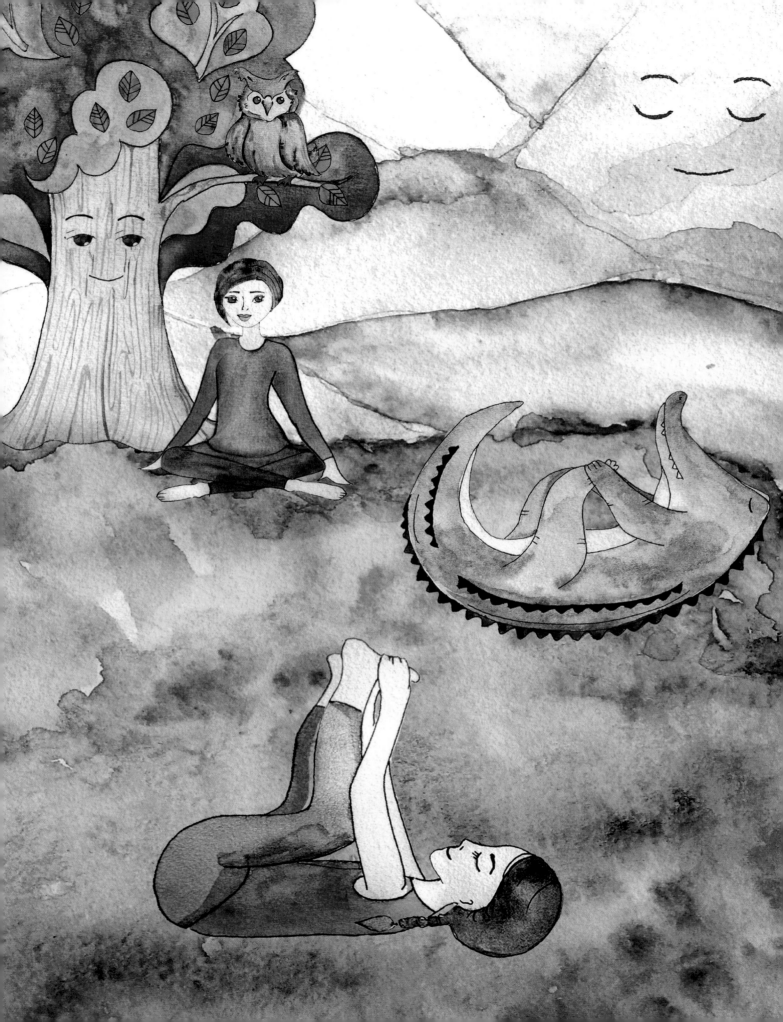

It really had been an exciting day in Nature. They spent a lot of time outside and she had learned so much, laughed a lot and even cried a little. Gina felt certain now that her mom would take her to the park more often. She fell back sleepily onto her Magical Mat, which appeared beneath her once more, and then she and her mom were quickly transported through Nature back to the City.

The butterfly was now clinging to Mom's shoulder again, holding on tightly as they circled through the misty clouds and the starry night sky. Gina didn't feel afraid now, but she still reached out for her mom's hand. This time Elizabeth accepted and held her hand gently. Gina felt calm, safe and loved.

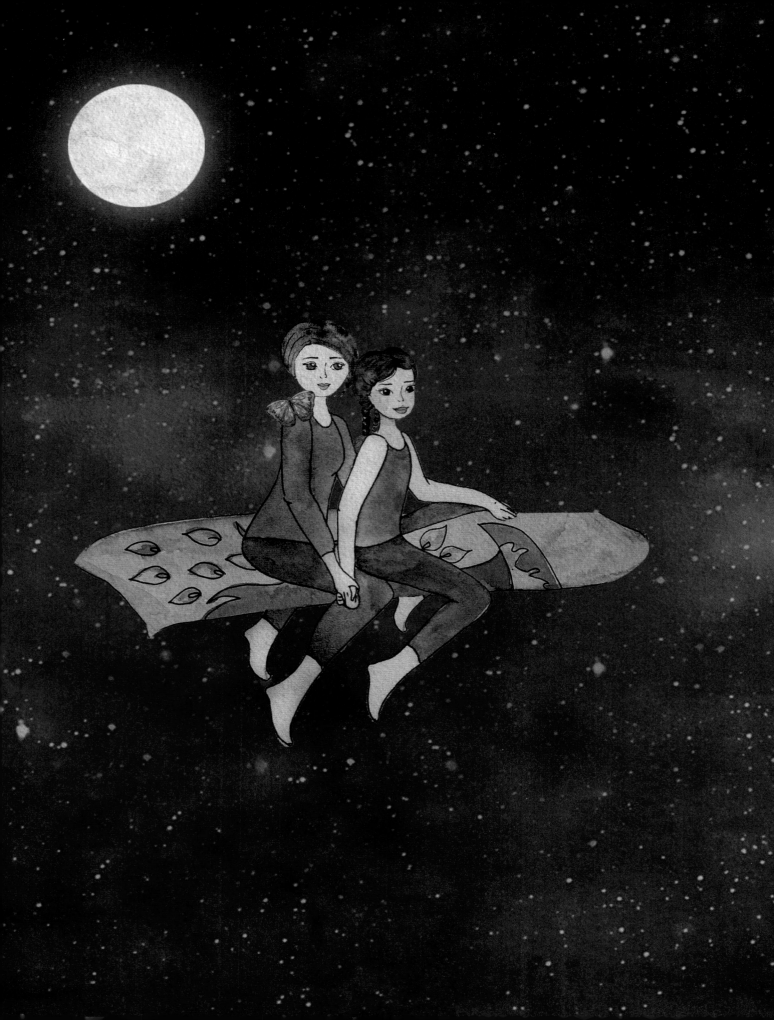

As if through a deep fog, Gina heard the familiar chime of the bell BG always rang at the end of class when the final resting pose was complete. She opened her eyes and saw that she was still connected to her mom, holding hands.

Gina blinked her eyes open slowly, letting her body come back into the space. She saw a familiar caterpillar crawling on the edge of her mom's mat. It was still a small, hairy caterpillar. This time she just took a big breath and observed its colors and herself. Nope! She didn't feel afraid!

Gina asked softly, "Mom, do you remember when we saw the butterfly in Nature and it flew back with us on your shoulder?"

But before her mom could answer, Gina knew something seemed strange. She saw BG sitting cross-legged in *Lotus Pose (Padmasana)* in the front of the room. She suddenly realized she must have been dreaming all along. Gina felt relieved to be grounded again and happy that her mom was present.

BG concluded, "As you bring awareness back into your body, remember today's intention. Notice how this one short class may have changed your body, mind and breathing. Today you showed bravery trying new poses and you've cultivated a sense of calm that you can take with you when you walk out the door. Remember, yoga is a continuous journey; the only thing that remains the same is that we are constantly changing and transforming. *Namaste.*"

They whole class answered, "*Namaste!*" and sang, "*Om Shanti, Shanti! Shanti! Peace! Peace! Peace!*" Yoga class ended just as usual, but Gina felt everything had changed. She was no longer afraid of the caterpillar, but it was much more than that. Gina felt strong, peaceful and sure of herself. She rolled up her mat and took her mom's hand once more. This time, Elizabeth gave her a gentle squeeze and smiled down at her daughter. Together they headed outside.

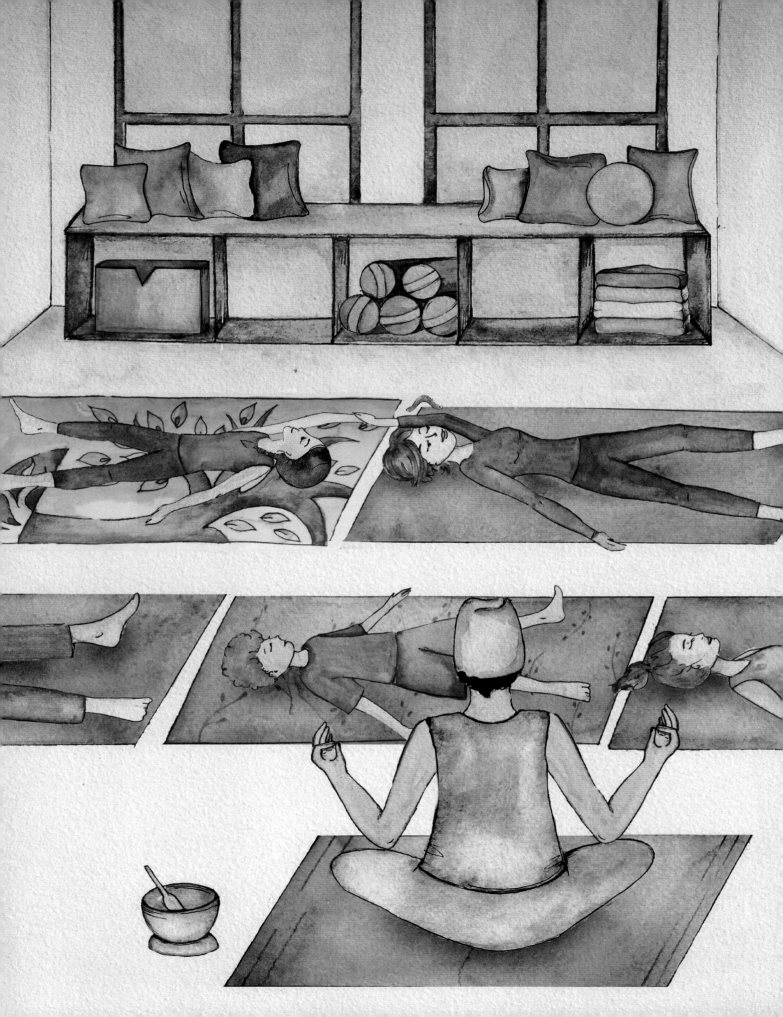

Although it was almost dinnertime, Gina and Elizabeth both noticed it was still light outside. As they started off towards home, Mom rolled down the windows. "It's good to let in the fresh air," she said. They heard a familiar "HOO, HOO!" ring out from the treetops, which seemed to call to them. Elizabeth looked at Gina lovingly and suddenly reached over to give her daughter's hand another squeeze. Instead of heading on their usual route home, she made a different turn. "How about a stroll through the park? This class reminded me of how much I miss being outside and watching you play."

It was true. Through the postures and deep meditation, she was reminded that self-care and time in nature are even more important than all the other things that kept her busy and trapped indoors. She was being the opposite of calm and brave and instead ran around full of fear, pressure and worry. All that negative energy Elizabeth was feeling was rubbing off on Gina, she could tell. After class, Elizabeth decided to make a conscious effort to do more things that her daughter wanted to do, things that would bring them both joy. She could sense the improvement and lightness already.

"Wow, Mom! It's just like BG's intention. You really got it this time! You seem so calm and content. Your attitude is changing just like the caterpillar transformed into a butterfly. You're like a new and improved mom! I like nature yoga mom best!"

Elizabeth laughed and smiled wide. "I like nature yoga mom best too!"

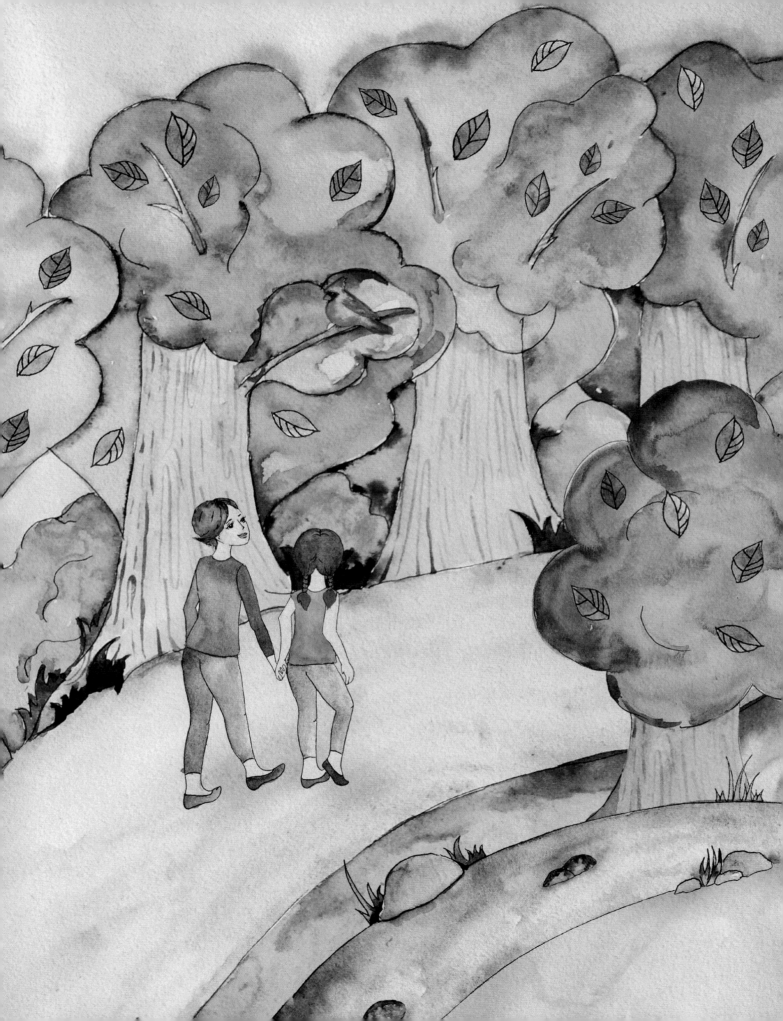

## Acknowledgments

I would like to take the opportunity to thank all the yoga teachers who either read my drafts, or provided greater insights into the practice of yoga from their perspectives. Of particular note, I would like to thank Lia Hulit who spent hours helping me do preliminary edits. I could not have done this without the help of my illustrator Alexandra Lotts. Her vision, her patience, her detail helped bring my words to life. Alexandra Lotts, is a self-taught illustrator, designer and photographer from Minsk, Belarus. She uses watercolor to inspire relaxation in people. Finally, I would like to thank the world-renowned publishing team of John Harricharan and Anita Bergen. A famous writer himself, John believed in my story from his very first review of the manuscript and his enthusiasm and guidance enabled me to publish this book.

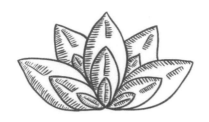

## About the Author

Traci Manuel is a business entrepreneur known for spending most of her days working in many time zones. As mentors, her parents continue to exemplify a work ethic that she came to emulate. Nevertheless, Traci came to yoga as a way to find both physical and emotional balance. Also, the practice of yoga has provided the missing piece to her life that she was seeking. She has met so many wonderful teachers and friends along this path. Although her yoga style has changed a lot over the years, even now, it continues to evolve. She also enjoys tending to her indoor plants, music, and looking at trees. Practic-ing the yoga philosophy of "Staying Present" she loves watching the ripples of the water as boats pass by, while she works at "being in the moment".